The Benefits of Smoking

Hale N. S. Mahon

<u>DEDICATION</u>

This book is dedicated to Frank and Lois Mahon.

INDRODUCTION

Most books regarding smoking are entitled something such as "The Disadvantages of Smoking" or "Why Smoking is a Terrible Vice from Hell", but in this book, we're trying a different tactic. This book is just a big list of all of the *good* things that can come from smoking.

.

www.ingramcontent.com/pod-product-compliance
Lightning Source LLC
Chambersburg PA
CBHW060500290526
45791CB00001B/204